A Wintry Walk

Keep Reading is an imprint of Proxy Care Publishing Ltd

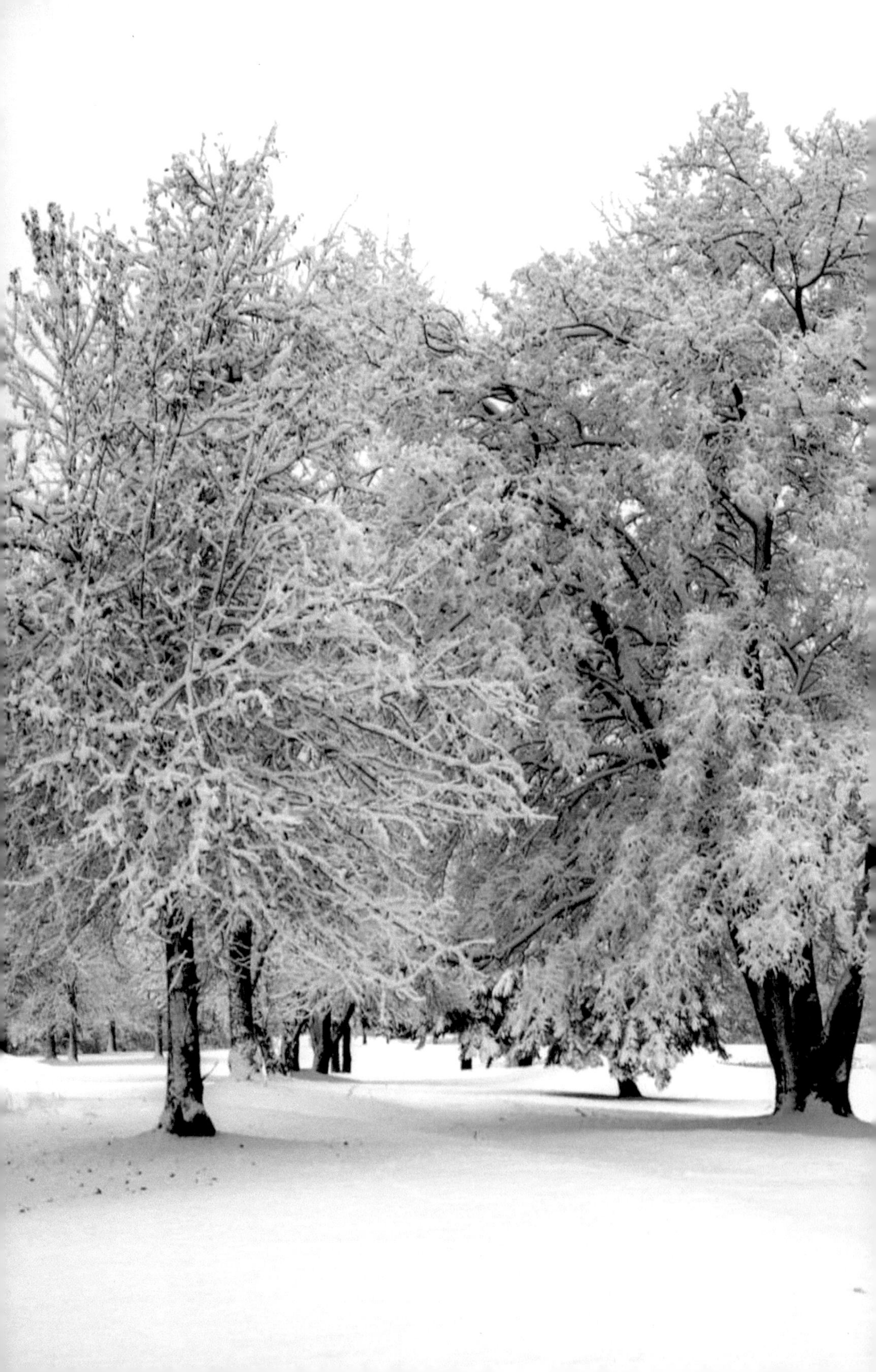

Chapter One

When the snow started falling the night before, a pang of excitement had filled Mary. She loved winter, at least for the first few months. The cold wore thin by March but when the leaves changed colors and fell off the trees in October and November, she anticipated the new season happily.

As soon as she woke in the early morning, she headed to the living room. Pushing back the heavy blue curtains of her window, Mary peered out at the transformed street. The beige sheers blocked her view, so she pushed those aside too. Now, she could see the narrow street covered in fresh whiteness. Big snowflakes still floated from the gray sky softly joining the others that had been gathering all night.

The first snow magically transformed the big maple trees surrounding her house. Their long rough branches, dark brown and twisted shined with three or four inches of pure, white crystals. Gathered at their base like a tumbled blanket, snow collected around the base of the trees covering the decaying, colored leaves with brightness.

Shivering slightly from the cold pushing against the glass panes, she smiled as she pulled her light blue, terry cloth bathrobe closer around her shoulders. Despite her scruffy brown slippers, her feet felt chilled too. It was one of the risks with having pine wood floors instead of carpeting, but she didn't mind. Her indoor heating system worked well so she was never too cold.

Walking over to the front door, she looked through the diamond shaped window to see her thermometer. Round and plastic, it had a green pine tree graphic against a white background and a round display showing the temperature. It was 18 degrees Fahrenheit and almost -8 degrees Celsius. Mary had grown up with Fahrenheit, but she still liked knowing both.

Despite the snow, it was warmer than it had been over the last ten days or so. Temperatures had dropped so low the news warned people to stay indoors as much as possible. It was too cold to snow, they said, but not anymore. The milder temperatures brought their first heavy snowfall of the winter season. They may have a white Christmas after all this year, Mary thought to herself, making her smile.

Leaving the curtains open, Mary fisted her hands inside the pockets of her robe to warm them as she walked through the living room then the dining room and into the kitchen.

Her living room was filled with matching tan and brown flowered couches and a brown recliner. A dark wood coffee table and two floor lamps rounded out the decor.

Her dining room contained a large, oval table with five chairs, and a matching China cabinet against the back wall. A bright basket of silk flowers sat in the center of the cherry wood dining table. She created the decoration the summer before after visiting a craft store. Choosing white baby's breath to thread in between coral peony, lavender lilacs, and blue hydrangea, she had been pleased with her project. Nestled in a tan willow basket, it brightened up the room nicely.

Once she reached her kitchen, she poured a cup of coffee from the old, glass decanter. The smoky nutty aroma filled her with a strong sense of warmth.

A few years earlier she had purchased a set of large, sage colored mugs from a flea market. They were just the right size with thick, rounded handles for her morning coffee. The heat of the cup felt good in her hands as she took her first, careful sip.

Taking her cup with her, she leaned forward to see the street and noticed the deep grooves from cars and trucks that had traveled since the snow began.

Drinking again and savoring the warm, slightly bitter taste, she decided she needed breakfast before she could venture out and genuinely enjoy the new weather.

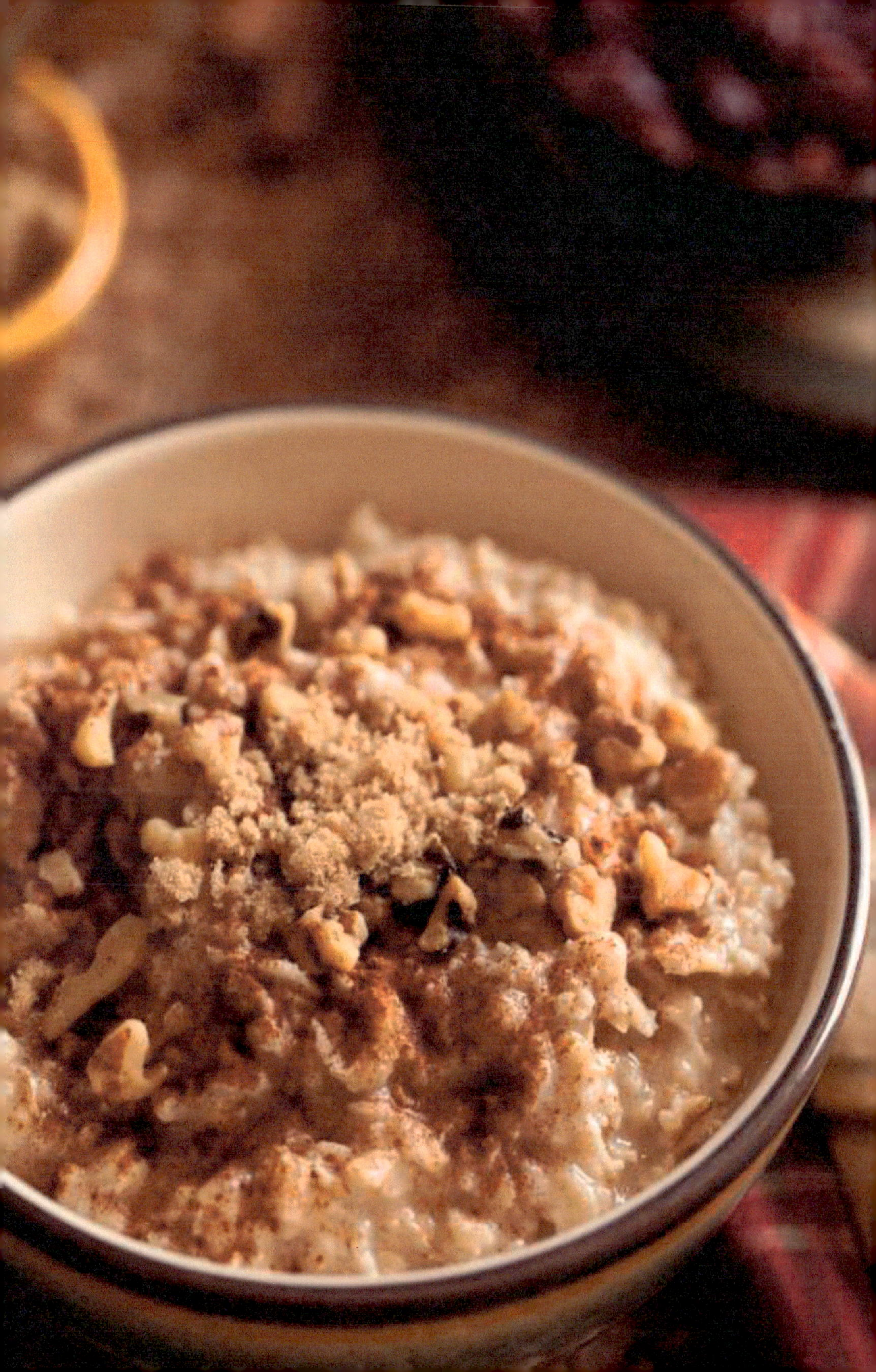

Chapter Two

Mary knew as soon as she saw the first flakes the night before that she would want to take a walk in the morning. There was nothing like the brisk cold and soft covering of fresh snow.

Mary opened the squeaky wood cabinet door and pulled a box of instant maple and brown sugar oatmeal down. Perfect for a chilly morning, she knew it would fill her up and sustain her until she returned home.

Opening the cardboard box, she plucked the small packet out. She chose her favorite ceramic bowl from another cupboard and set it on the counter with a light clunk. The oatmeal flakes fell into the bowl, smelling sweet with the hint of maple and apple.

Mary took a small saucepan from the cupboard next to the stove and filled it with water. The saucepan was old and had been part of a gold set she had used until the handles grew weak and the deep scratches made the other pieces useless.

She pushed the cold metal handle of the single faucet up allowing cool water to flow, enjoying the plunk as it hit the saucepan and filled.

Once she had enough for her oatmeal, she shut off the water then went to the stove. Turning the plastic knob on the front, it flamed with a small whoosh and then she placed the saucepan on the burner.

While the water heated, she returned to the kitchen window to watch the plump snowflakes plummet slowly to the ground and on the roof tops and tree branches, adding a fresh layer to the three or four inches already accumulated.

Hearing the water boiling, Mary reluctantly left the window. Gripping the hard, plastic handle in one hand, she turned the heat off with the other, then poured the bubbling liquid into her bowl. Opening the utensil drawer with a hard yank because it tended to stick, she took out a metal spoon. She topped the oatmeal off with some chopped walnuts and brown sugar from two small canisters she had resting on the counter.

The sweet maple aroma drifted from the bowl as she stirred, and her stomach growled in anticipation. Carefully, picking up the warm bowl and her cup of coffee, she carried both back to the living room so she could watch the snow while she enjoyed her breakfast.

Settling into the deep cushion of her couch, she took a long drink of coffee. It was cooling and nearly perfect temperature. As she looked out, she noticed her neighbor from across the street, propping a red snow shovel by his back door.

It was too soon to start clearing the walkways yet. He would need to wait until the snow stopped. Mary intended to retrieve her shovel when she returned from her walk.

Growing excited to be outside, Mary barely noticed the warm, sweet taste of the oatmeal. She was fascinated with the sight of some brown and white birds hopping from the Franklins' Gem bush lining her porch to the snowy front yard.

They seemed to be chattering to each other while they took short flights from the bush to the yard. Mary knew they would eventually find her red and yellow bird feeder hanging in the back yard.

Her spoon clattered against glass, Mary looked down to find her bowl mostly empty. She popped up, it was time to get dressed and head out into the beautifully decorated morning.

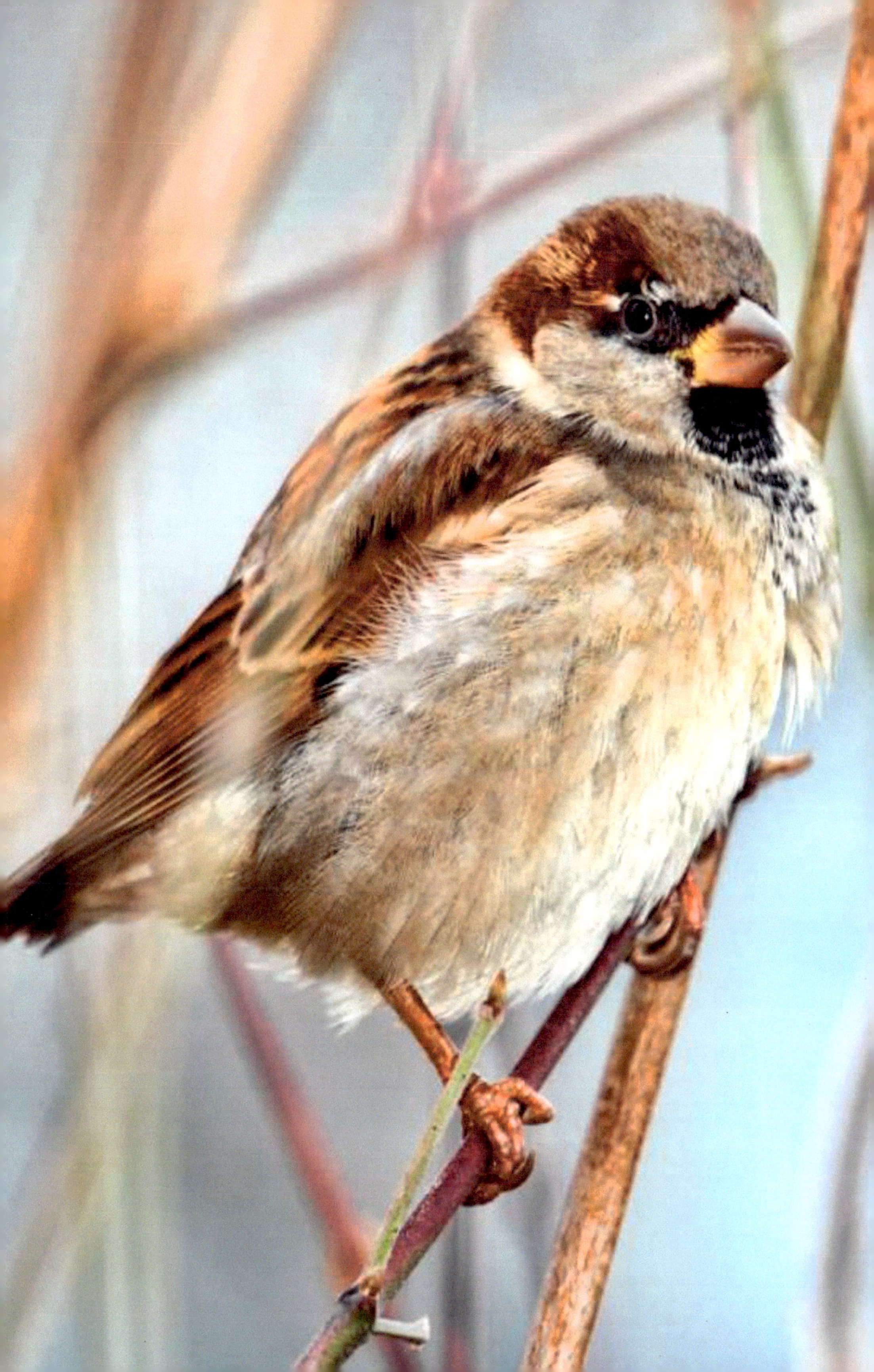

Chapter Three

Having showered the night before, she just needed to choose the right clothes to venture into the cold. Going into her bedroom, Mary took a moment to make the bed.

She pulled the cream-colored sheets up followed by the heavy brown comforter. After dropping her pillows on top, she straightened some of the wrinkles.

With that chore done, Mary walked into her closet and tugged a pair of cozy blue pants off the white plastic hanger. Then she found a soft, pink sweatshirt with the white emblem of a cruise ship on the front. She bought it after taking a dinner cruise. Taking that off the hanger, she tossed both pieces on to her bed.

Next, she chose a long sleeved, white cotton top to wear beneath the sweatshirt.

Going to her tall, teal painted dresser, she opened the top drawer. After rummaging through the contents, she found a heavy pair of pink wool socks to wear under her brown, winter boots. The boots had been a splurge last winter, but she loved the way they hugged her feet and kept them warm. Even her toes stayed toasty and dry inside.

Once she was dressed in her warmest clothes, she slid the boots on. They were light brown leather with darker brown laces and jagged rubber treads. They came up just passed her ankles. She sat on the bed and tightened the laces, enjoying the snug feeling and glad to have them for her walk.

After brushing her hair and teeth, Mary was ready to brave the frigid day.

The living room closet stored all her coats, jackets, and winter ware. She had installed some wooden shelves where she could keep mittens, gloves, and hats as well as summer things like colorful gardening gloves and bandanas.

She picked a knitted toque that would cover her ears and her irrepressible brown curls. The cap was pink and fuzzy and matched her mittens. Glancing at the long, knit scarf folded on the shelf she wondered if she would need it. It was black with squares of pink. Soft and warm, she thought it might be too warm and didn't know if she wanted to wear it. After a moment's consideration, she decided she'd store it inside her purse, so she'd have it if needed.

Returning to the kitchen, Mary took a short grocery list off the refrigerator. The magnet holding the narrow blue paper was strong and she had to pluck it off to retrieve the list. The magnet was shaped like a bear and colored black with dark eyes, the word “Yellowstone” was printed in yellow across its belly.

She stashed the paper in the back pocket of her pants, checked the stove to be sure she had turned it off and grabbed her purse from the kitchen counter.

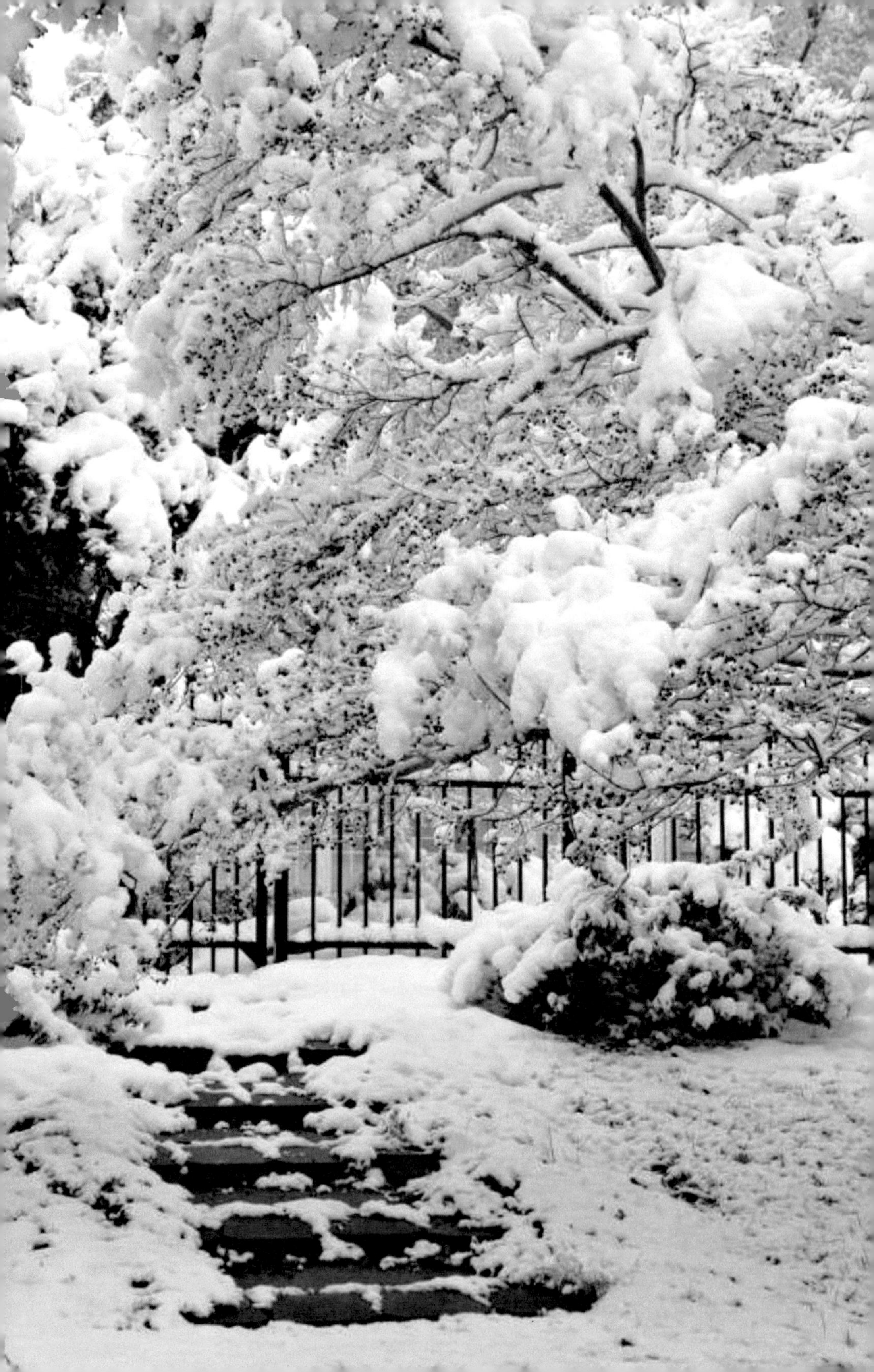

Chapter Four

Mary opened the heavy front door and caught her breath as the brisk morning met her. She turned the cold, metal handle on the storm door and pushed it free. Another blast of winter blew against her, and she couldn't keep the smile off her face.

Taking a shallow breath, she welcomed the chill into her lungs.

Looking out across her wide front porch, the silence, like a peaceful friend surrounded her. It seemed almost dreamlike as she turned from one view to the next, not hearing any sounds of people or machinery. Even the breeze moved quietly, sending mists of new snow into the air.

Fat wet flakes continued tumbling to the ground, caught in the gentle wind, twisting, and turning aimlessly from the awakening white sky.

She loved this moment, the bright white, almost painful to behold and the endless quiet. It seemed as if no one existed but her and there was such peace in the feeling.

Pulling her pink hat down further, she moved over the planks of wood towards the cement steps leading to the world outside her door. The covered roof of the porch kept most of the flakes away, but a thin layer lay in streaks. On the railings, a few inches or so of snow had accumulated so she playfully pushed it off, enjoying the way it plunked towards the ground.

With careful steps in case there was hidden ice, she used the old narrow handrail to descend. She took the last step to the cement walkway and looked towards the sky. Snowflakes kissed her cheeks and eyes. She stuck her tongue out like a child and felt the cold-water touch down. Tasteless and frigid, it still felt wonderful.

She took another moment to scan her empty neighborhood noticing the light smell of firewood burning as chimneys released spirals of smoke into the air. Not for the first time, she wished her house came equipped with a fireplace knowing it would be homey and warm.

Tugging on her soft, warm mittens, she started her stroll to the store. She pulled the long strap of her leather bag further up her shoulder and secured it with one hand.

Mary closed her eyes and turned her face upward again allowing the heavy wet flakes to land on her nose and lips. She shivered but the sensation felt good.

"All right," she said softly, not wanting to break the frigid silence. "Time to get a move on."

Her boots pushed through the fluffy layer of snow that had fallen. She enjoyed creating the first footsteps on the snow-covered sidewalk. It reminded her of leaving footprints in the sand, only it was her boot prints she saw in the snow.

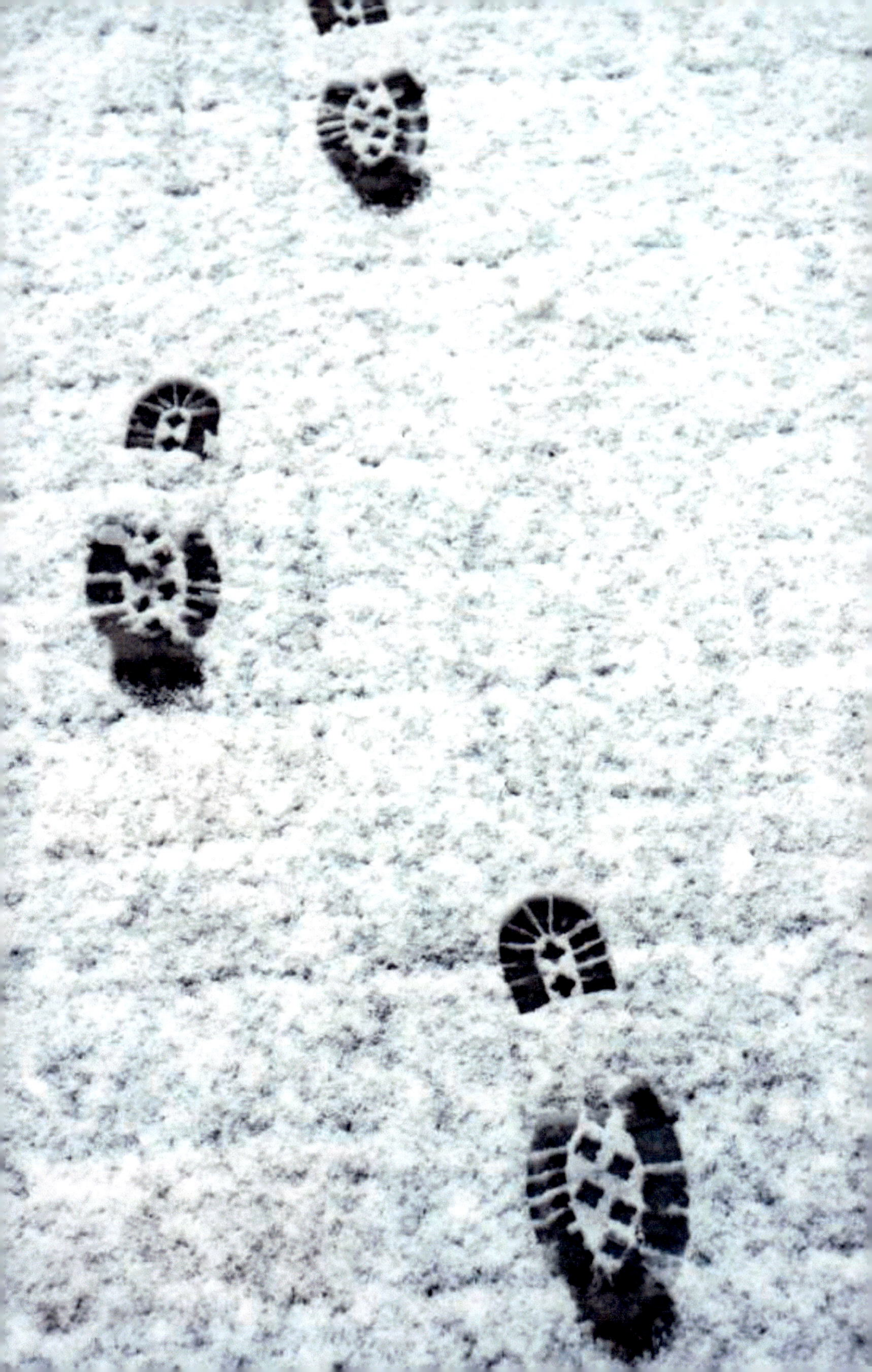

Chapter Five

About halfway down the block, Mary turned around to look at the impressions of her boots in the previously untouched snow. She knew it wouldn't be long before others trod along her path but for the moment it was fun to see the solitude of just two feet leaving a trail.

The small park on the other side of the street was not a short cut to the store but it was beautiful in all sorts of weather. Maple and elm trees circled the perimeter providing a barrier to the street, and narrow trees with ashy trunks and orange leaves in the summer, lined the footpaths.

Mary crossed the street, after a car passed, but just the one. Little traffic ventured on to the small street.

The road was more slippery than the sidewalk and she gasped when her right foot hit an icy spot and she slid forward, arms pinwheeling to regain her balance. When she slid to a stop, still standing, she giggled softly despite her pounding heart.

"You're going to break your neck," she chided herself but laughed about it anyway.

Confident she was steady again, Mary carefully walked through the snow and on to the walking path that hadn't been shoveled.

The heavy snow had stopped, replaced by light flurries fluttering on the breeze.

As she entered the center of the park, it was like the world had suddenly been plunged into a fairy tale. She marveled at the way the snow sparkled under the streetlamps. A bright red cardinal swooped down and then up again to land on the top of the light.

The benches, painted green, were barely visible under the thick layer of snow. And no one sat on them. A young couple stood close by, speaking softly to each other. And Mary noted they were the first people she had seen since spying her neighbor from her living room window.

The girl wore a dark blue, nylon coat that hung to the top of her black pants. Her hands were covered in black gloves and a navy scarf was wrapped around her neck. Light blonde hair spilled over her shoulders. The boy used his bare hands to gesture while he spoke. Mary could see his knuckles and fingers were red from the cold. He wore only a red hoodie emblazoned with the NYU logo and blue jeans. Just the sight of him gave Mary a shiver up her spine. Oh, to be young again, Mary thought, remembering when the cold didn't worry her as much.

If they noticed Mary passing, they didn't show it but, that was okay. Mary was enjoying her early morning solitude.

Laying heavily on bowing tree branches along the path, a sudden wind blew the snow into a swirling mass that seemed to disappear into the air. Clamping her mittened hands over her cap with a dull clumping sound, she prevented it from blowing away too.

Mary pulled her purse back up on to her shoulder and noticed her fingers starting to grow cold. She slid them into her coat pocket for protection and took a deep breath. Unconsciously she had stiffened against the cold, and she knew from experience that keeping her body relaxed was a much better way to handle the chilly morning.

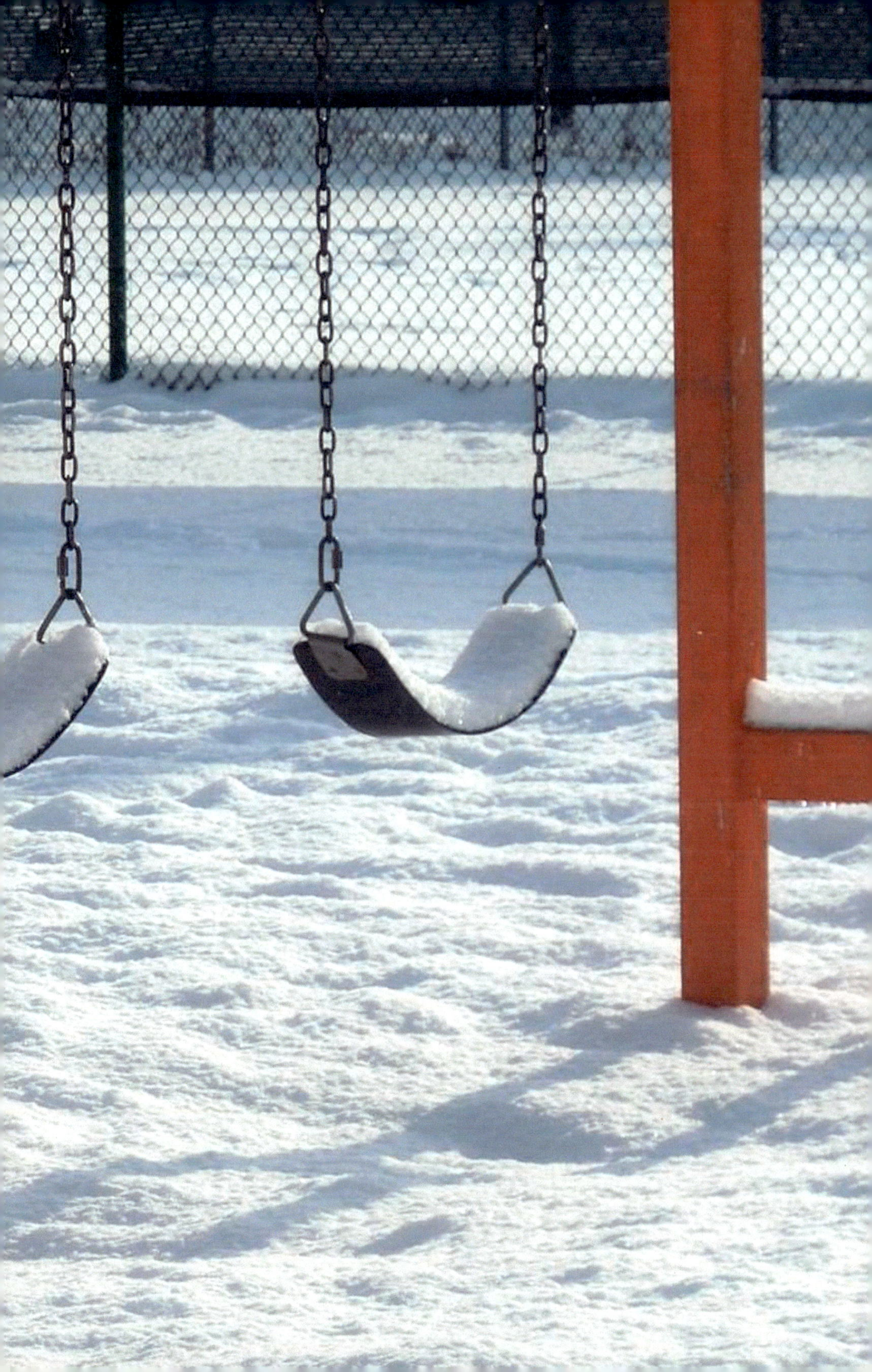

Chapter Six

As Mary reached the center of the park, she decided to continue straight and pass the playground. It was probably too cold for young children to climb on the blue and red plastic jungle gym or the swings with their metal chains and rubber seats.

Traveling slowly as the wind pushed back against her, Mary found she was right. The playground was empty with snow heaped on every surface. The stark cold and barren equipment had an almost eerie quality in the silence.

Then as she looked down the narrow walkway, she spotted a family tossing snowballs at each other. Two young children, bundled tightly in heavy coats, mittens and hats ran this way and that, trying to make ammunition while the parents, also darting around threw lightly packed snowballs. Everyone was laughing while they chased each other, and the sound was a musical interruption to the quiet.

Mary laughed when one of the children made a wild throw and it zinged past her ear. The mother stopped, with a horrified expression. The father froze too and one of the kids took advantage to fling a snowball and hit him in the chest with a splat.

"I'm so sorry," the mother said.

"Not at all," Mary said. "I don't know if you saw it but there's usually a drink stand with hot chocolate just down the path on the left."

“We didn’t see it. Thank you so much. The girls will love that.”

“Have fun,” Mary said, her heart lifting at the sight of the small group having such a good time together.

Continuing her walk through the park, Mary flexed her fingers inside her coat to warm them. She spotted a bushy tailed squirrel standing up on its back legs and sniffing the air before darting across the path, and up the narrow tree trunk. Mary followed it with her eyes and was pleased to see another one with fluffy white and brown fur and a busy nose. Both squirrels sunk a few inches into the snow drift on the branch.

A couple of boys pulling sleds behind them distracted her from the squirrels. The crunching of their footsteps and the scraping sound of the sleds caught her attention.

She guessed that school must have declared a snow day.

The sleds were round and silver with heavy cords that the boys clutched in their hands. From the grooves and scratches in the metal it looked like they had been used often.

One of the boys glanced up at her, smiled lightly and then put his head back down as they trudged their way towards whatever mammoth hill they could find.

Mary carefully moved up a small rise. Stepping gingerly to avoid slippery spots she reached the small summit and gasped softly.

The round pond had frozen over. Normally, a fishing spot in the spring and summer, it was now frozen solid. And people had somehow, magically known.

Skaters danced along the surface. Some graceful with arms extended, legs moving smoothly as they glided. Others more tentative, clunking against the ice with their arms waving for balance. There were adults holding the hands of little ones scooting one step at a time, and teenagers chasing each other laughing and hollering.

The scene was framed under the beautiful snow falling across them, landing on knit hats of all colors. Snowflakes, swirled in the wind, dropping with an almost audible plunk.

Snowbanks, more than four feet tall, lined the edges of the pond. Someone had shoveled to clear the ice and children ran along the top, sliding down then climbing to slide again. Their laughter rang out like faint chimes across the distance.

Mary clapped, her hands thudding softly because of the mittens, when a lovely female skater turned into a spinning top. With great elegance, she hugged her waist and spun so quickly it was almost dizzying to watch. As she slowed to a stop, Mary noticed several other skaters had stopped to clap too.

Wanting to stay and watch, Mary thought about the short grocery list and her chilled body. While her boots had maintained warm dry feet, the rest of her was cold and getting damp.

She considered the hot coffee waiting inside the store and decided she could warm up, get the few things she needed and return, armed with the steaming liquid, and perhaps a warm salty pretzel from the bakery.

Glad she had packed the multi-colored scarf in her purse, Mary knew she could use it for extra comfort when she came back out.

There were benches around the amateur rink to sit on, and a beautiful winter day to still enjoy.

Happy with her decision, Mary hesitated for another moment to watch the talented skater launch into another spin, this time with one foot lifted above the ice and her arms raised gracefully above her head. Her white skates were bright against her black tights, and her floral skirt whirled as she spun, it was dazzling to see. Clapping again, as the girl whooshed to a stop, Mary forced herself to get moving so she could finish her errand and return.

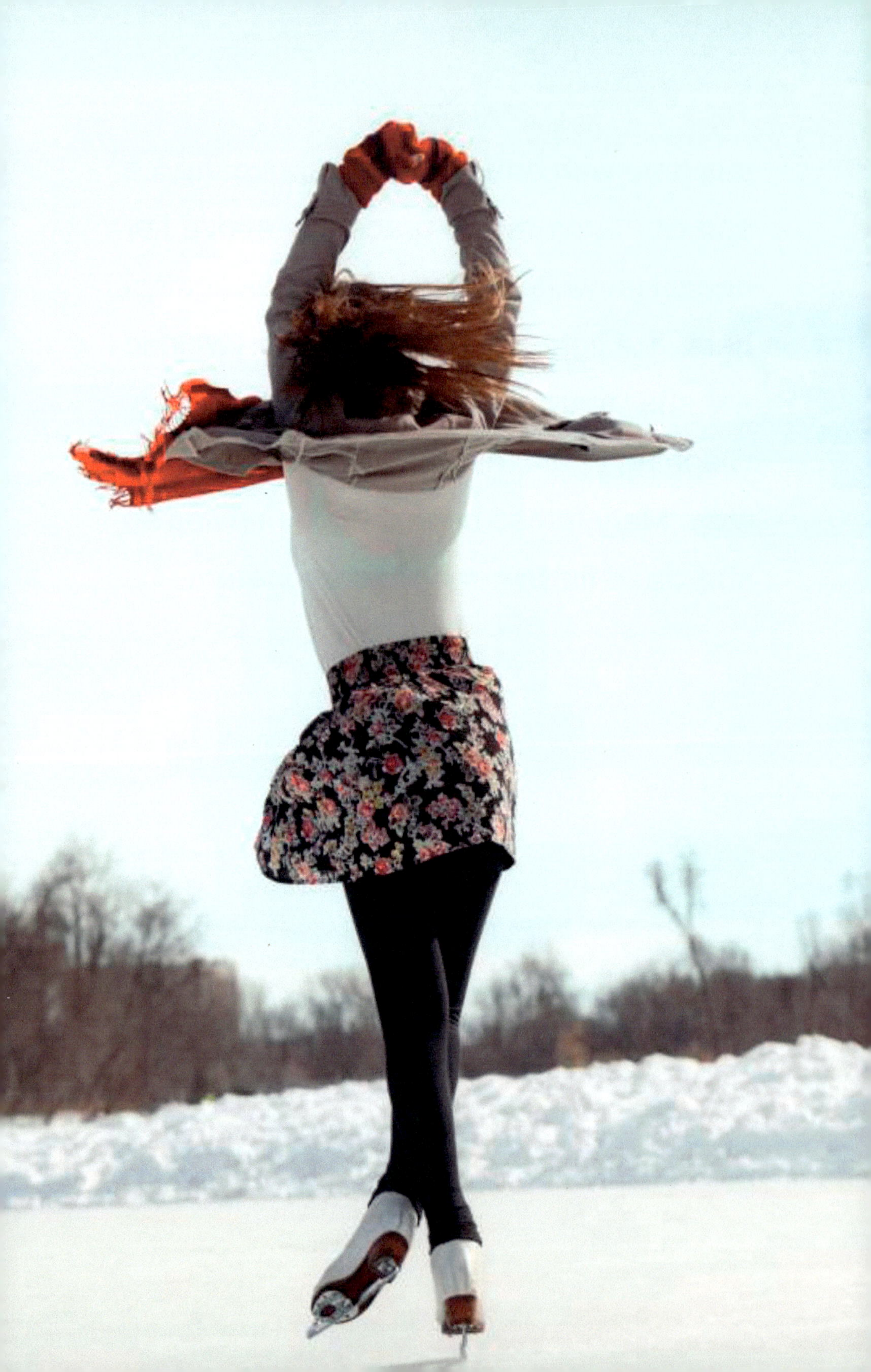

Chapter Seven

As Mary reached the sidewalk that edged along the park, she stepped out of the fairy tale and began to travel the final block towards her destination. The cement squares beneath her feet were still covered in fresh delicate snow. Her perfect footprints followed her path like a casted shadow. There were several other sets of footprints along the sidewalk now. Deep waffle imprints mixed with shallower decorative markings that probably belonged to sneakers shuffled across the street. She even spotted some peg holes that likely meant a woman in heels had trod across the new snow.

The people, whoever they were, had gone on with their days leaving nothing but prints to show they had passed by.

From where she stood, Mary could see the orange glowing lights of the grocery store like a beacon against the heavily clouded sky. Vaguely looking forward to escaping the cold for a few minutes, she anticipated buying a chocolate-flavored coffee to drink on the walk back to the pond. Sweet and hot, it would warm her body. She could practically feel the heat sliding down her throat and into her belly.

Happy with the idea, Mary walked more quickly towards the store, rubbing her arms. The snow fall had never completely stopped, and it was starting to fall harder.

The wind had picked up too and she shivered despite her coat and winter gear.

Stepping on another icy patch, she caught herself again. It wasn't as dramatic as the first time, but she had to grab the trunk of an elm tree to steady herself. The bark felt rough against her mittens. She hung on for a moment, laughing again and pressing her forehead against the cold wood.

"You all right, lady?" A voice asked and Mary looked up to see a red pickup pulled to the side of the road. A man, dark haired and bearded, maybe college aged, had rolled down the passenger window.

"Yes, thank you so much," she answered, grinning. She loved living in a small town where people were kind to each other.

"Do you need any help?" He asked.

"No, no, I'm quite all right, thank you. Just enjoying this beautiful snow."

The man looked uncertain as he said, "Okay, well, have a nice day."

"You too," she said.

He rolled up the automatic window, put on his blinker and drove off.

Mary let go of the tree and carefully returned to the sidewalk. She was still giggling as she made her way to the store.

At the edge of the grocery store parking lot, Mary spied three girls. Two were quite young and wearing matching red coats. The third girl, wearing a white coat with black snowpants, was probably an early teen. The little ones lay in the snow on either side of the older one and they were all furiously flapping their arms and legs back and forth, sending chilly mists into the sky.

When they stopped moving, the older girl warned them to be careful as they stood up.

“Don’t mess up the angels,” she said.

The younger ones moved slowly, trying their best not to leave any prints from hands or feet.

Mary couldn’t hide her smile as she saw the joy spreading across their faces as the girls looked down on their creations.

It was another lovely moment from a wintery walk filled with all the joys of winter.

She carefully walked by the girls, stepping from the street sidewalk into the parking lot. The aroma of freshly baked bread drifted from the store, and she anticipated the coffee and pretzel waiting for her inside.

Feeling satisfied with the morning, Mary knew there was nothing like the first big snow of the season and she was embracing it and enjoying every moment of her walk. It might be another year before she could savor it again but, it was always magical and worth the wait.

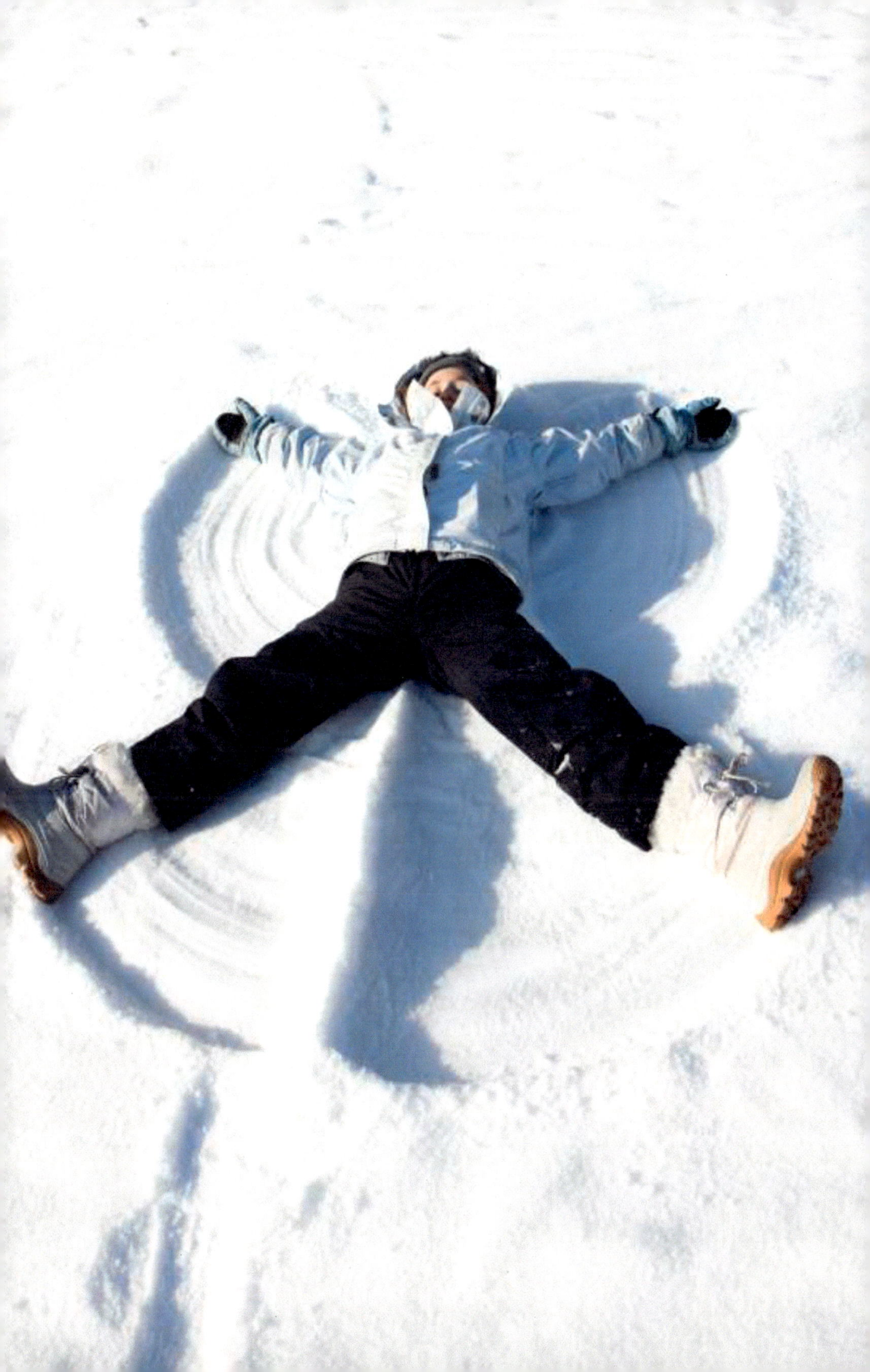

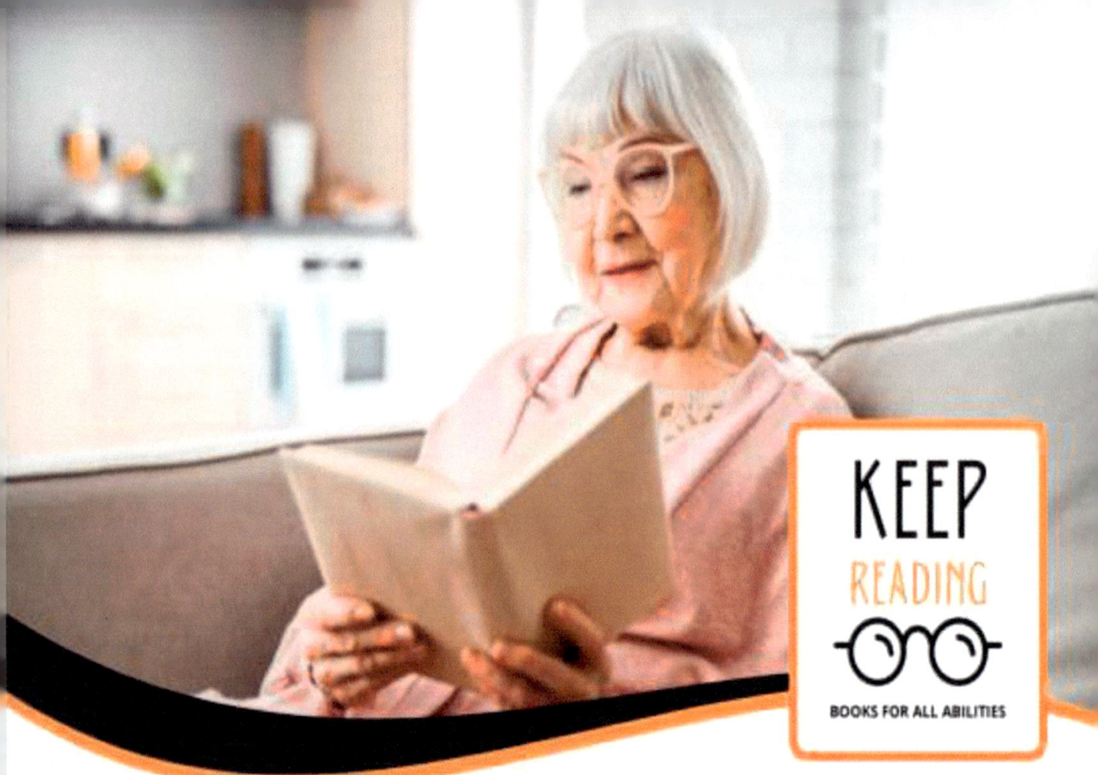

TRY MORE BOOKS BY KEEP READING

ARE YOU AT THE RIGHT KEEP READING LEVEL??

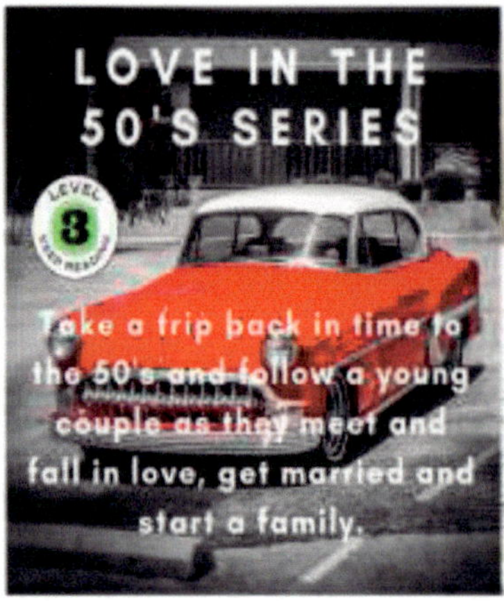

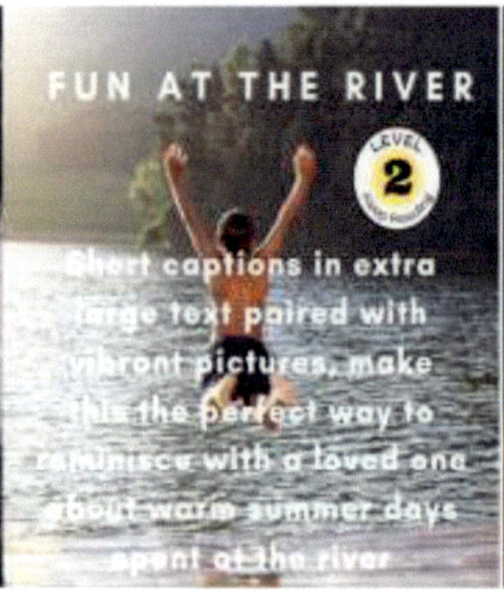

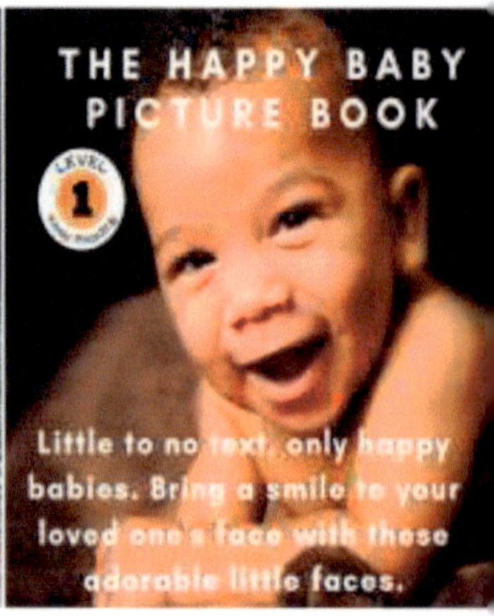

www.keepreading.ca

Made in the USA
Monee, IL
05 November 2026

67379945R00031